Know Your Nuts:

Top healthiest nut to consume

By

Lois R. Chappell

DISCLAIMER

Before this document is duplicated or reproduced in any manner, the publisher's consent must be gained. Therefore, the content within can neither be stored electronically, transferred, nor kept in a database. Neither in part nor full can the document be copied, scanned, faxed or retained without approval from the publisher or creator.

DEDICATION

This book is dedicated to God Almighty first and foremost, to my mother, Mrs. Veronica, our mother earth for the uncompensated gift of nature, and everyone who believes in nature.

TABLE OF CONTENT

Chapter 7:

TIPS FOR STORING NUTS

INTRODUCTION

Nuts are nature's way of teaching us that awesome things come in small packages. These bite-size nutritional powerhouses contain heart-healthy fats, protein, vitamins, and minerals.

Nuts have several health benefits, from supporting a healthy heart to maybe fighting against cancer. However, they are high in nutrients and contain heart-healthy fats; nuts have many benefits and can be ingested daily.

Some people might assume they're on a low-calorie diet, but that's false. In reality, nuts are nutrient-packed and work as terrific snacks if you are attempting to reduce weight.

If you are not allergic to nuts, it is entirely acceptable to eat a small handful of nuts every day (be sure to check for shriveling or blemishes, which can be an indication your nuts have gone wrong) .

If you have specific health issues, such as high blood pressure and diabetes, you may choose unsalted nuts over salted or flavored ones. Like with other food, consuming nuts in moderate amounts gives lots of positive health benefits.

They're excellent for snacking as they are, but you can also use them in dishes like Cranberry-Almond Energy Balls, Cherry-Chocolate Chip Granola Bars, or

Baked Banana-Nut Oatmeal Cups to shake up your routine.

In this book, you will discover which nut is packed with high protein, has the lowest fat and calorie content, how it can be incorporated into diets including tips on how to preserve them for the long term. I have picked up the 10 healthiest nuts to graze on, with reliable nutritional information on how to enjoy them in your diet.

CHAPTER 1

NUTS AND SEEDS

Is eating nuts healthy for you?

Nuts and seeds are foods rich in nutrients and offer a wide range of advantages to one's health. These are beautiful places to get your fill of fiber, protein, healthy fats, and vitamins and minerals.

Almonds, walnuts, pistachios, cashews, peanuts, pumpkin seeds, chia seeds, and flaxseeds are among the most prevalent nuts and seeds. Walnuts are also quite popular.

It has been found that those who include nut and seed consumption as part of a balanced diet had a lower chance of developing cardiovascular disease, diabetes, and some types of cancer.

They also offer several benefits for the brain's health, including improving cognitive function and reducing the risk of cognitive decline associated with aging.

However, it is essential to remember that nuts and seeds have many calories; hence, it is necessary to take them in moderation to maintain a healthy and well-balanced diet. If you suffer from a nut allergy, you must avoid nuts at all costs and talk to a doctor or other qualified medical practitioner about possible substitutions.

Nuts are an excellent source of healthy fats, vitamins, and minerals, and they also include protein. Yet, which of these options is the most beneficial?

In the United Kingdom, we eat an all-time high quantity of nuts. One possible explanation for this trend is the increased focus on health and plant-based diets. The days are long gone when consumers have to decide between buying salted or dry-roasted peanuts.

The variety of nut products, such as whole nuts, nut butter, and nut milk, as well as other nut-based foods, has expanded substantially during the past several decades.

You may have thought that nuts are unhealthy due to their high-fat content, but this is only part of the story. Nuts are a nutrient-dense food providing fiber, protein, vitamins, minerals, and other essential micronutrients.

Consuming nuts may lower one's chance of developing cardiovascular and circulatory illnesses. It has also been suggested as a more sustainable method for our world that, rather than eating meat and dairy products, people should consume nuts and pulses as their primary protein sources.

Some research has also shown that people who consume nuts regularly have a lower risk of suffering a heart attack or passing away from one. In addition, eating nuts has been shown to reduce cholesterol and triglyceride levels in the blood.

Take, for instance: One of the unique advantages of walnuts is that they contain antioxidants. Antioxidants, such as polyphenols, can nullify the effects of free radicals in the body, leading to less damage to cells.

 Free radicals are molecules prone to instability and can raise the disease risk. Walnuts, which are great for vegans and people who eat meat because of their superior capacity to combat free radicals, have been the subject of extensive research

CHAPTER 2

WHY DO WE EAT NUTS?

The benefits of nuts to one's health:

Consuming a wide variety of nuts is crucial since each type of nut has a unique set of health advantages. Because of their high-calorie content, nuts should be consumed in moderation.

There are several reasons why nuts are included on practically every best-of list for healthy snacks.

To begin, they are simple to transport in a bag if you are going somewhere or to store in a drawer or pantry if you want to have them on hand. In addition to protein and other minerals, all nuts have fiber, which helps lower cholesterol and makes you feel full for a more extended period, assisting you in eating less.

Your diet can be packed with complete protein, fiber, unsaturated fats, and essential vitamins and minerals by including just a small handful of them. Several significant health benefits have been associated with the consumption of nuts.

In addition to containing "good" fats that may lower your LDL or "bad" cholesterol and triglyceride levels, most nuts also contain omega-3 fatty acids and vitamin E, which may help prevent plaque buildup in the arteries. "Good" fats may lower your LDL or "bad" cholesterol and triglyceride levels.

In a previous study, researchers discovered that people who reported eating the most nuts had a roughly 35 percent lower risk of coronary heart disease than those who ate fewer nuts. This finding was compared to individuals who ate fewer nuts.

According to another body of research, increased nut consumption among the 15,467 older women who participated in the Nurses' Health Study over six years was associated with the participants' improved general cognition. People who reported eating nuts more regularly had a longer life expectancy than those who ate nuts less frequently. According to the findings of another study that involved nearly 120,000 participants and was partially funded by the International Tree Nut Council Nutrition

Research and Education Foundation, agrees to the fact that people who eat more nuts have extended lifespan.

Thus, you must include nuts in your daily snack rotation to ensure you get all the significant disease-fighting nutrients that may help protect your heart, lower your cholesterol, and have various other health benefits.

The following list provides the top ten justifications for using nuts in one's diet.

1. Loaded with many essential nutrients

As was mentioned, this is one of the primary arguments favoring including nuts in one's diet, which is strongly recommended. They are brimming with vitamins, calcium, iron, potassium, magnesium, manganese, protein, fiber, and a wide variety of other nutrients essential to the body's ability to function correctly.

2. Assists the body in the process of absorbing nutrients

Nuts include a high proportion of heart-healthy fats. Which often gives them a bad name and may make them appear unsuited for a diet to aid in weight loss. Despite this, however, it is essential for our bodies to consume healthy fats. Unsaturated fats are beneficial to our health and assist our bodies in absorbing vitamins and other nutrients from the food we eat.

3. Rich in antioxidative properties

Antioxidant properties are found in abundance in nuts. Antioxidants are substances that assist in the elimination of numerous toxins that can be found in our bodies. Antioxidants help eliminate free radicals from our bodies by removing harmful radicals from the environment.

4. Aids digestion

Dried fruits enhance our digestion. Nuts are widely regarded as a beneficial dietary inclusion for individuals with poor gut health. They contain a high proportion of fiber. Fiber's presence considerably aids the transportation of our food through our digestive tract in our diet.

5. Ensures a restful night's sleep

Suppose you are still hungry after or before bedtime; nuts like almonds and walnuts make excellent post-dinner snacks. Consuming nuts triggers the production of a variety of feel-good hormones. It has been established that feel-good hormones like serotonin contribute to higher sleep quality.

6. Nuts have been shown to promote several functions in the heart, which contributes to improved heart health. They assist in improving blood circulation in addition to many other aspects. In addition to this, several studies have shown that making nuts a regular part of your diet will help lower your chances of having a form of heart disease that is chronic. These may also lessen the likelihood that you may have a heart attack.

7. Contributes to weight loss

Contrary to the widespread notion, nuts are an excellent complement to a diet that aims to reduce one's body fat percentage. They include a lot of protein, making the metabolism go much faster. In addition, they are an excellent replacement for unhealthy snacks and help you feel filled for a more extended period.

8. Reduces levels of cholesterol

It has been demonstrated that nuts can lower our bodies' cholesterol levels, known as "bad" cholesterol. Nuts have been shown to inhibit the body's uptake of the "bad" kind of cholesterol. They lessen the desire to eat unhealthy snacks and satisfy cravings. This can make it easier for you to steer clear of cholesterol-rich meals.

9. Versatile

Consuming the same meals day in and day out takes a lot of work. Nuts, in contrast to many other healthful foods, are highly versatile. They can be consumed naturally, made into milk, used as a garnish, and for various uses. Because of this, including them in one's diet is possible and relatively simple.

10. It helps the immune system.

Nuts are a great immune system booster due to their high concentration of minerals and antioxidants. Nuts are an effective weapon against free radicals in the environment and may even aid conditions that were already present to improve their symptoms.

CHAPTER 3

TOP HEALTHIEST NUT:

with verified nutritional data on how to incorporate them into your diet

A nut is a straightforward dry fruit with one or two edible kernels enclosed in a tough shell. According to a study, including nuts regularly in a balanced diet can help us maintain a healthy weight and fend off chronic illnesses (such as heart disease and diabetes).

The top healthy nut choices include almonds, Brazil nuts, cashew nuts, hazelnuts, macadamias, pecans, pine nuts, pistachios, walnuts, and chestnuts.

The benefits each nut can have on your health are listed below:

1. Walnuts:

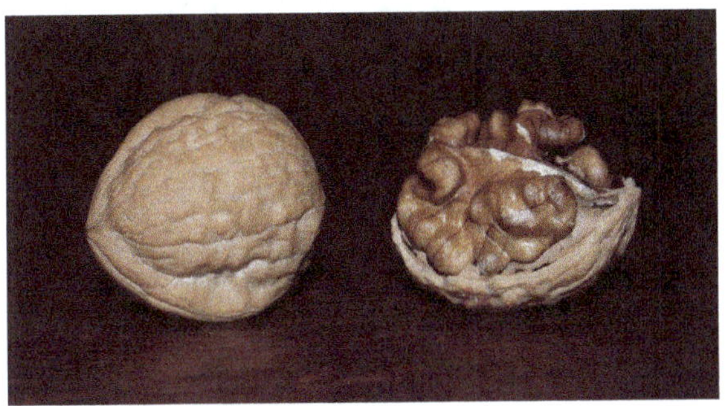

Fight Inflammation and Are Rich in Antioxidants.

Consuming a daily intake of walnuts can enhance cognitive performance and lower the risk of dementia-related conditions such as cardiovascular disease, depression, and type 2 diabetes.

Walnuts offer 'good-for-you' fats like all nuts do; in this case, they are primarily polyunsaturated fats (PUFAs). In fact, of all edible plants, walnuts have the highest concentration of alpha lipoic acid (ALA), a short-chain omega-3 essential fatty acid, making them a highly beneficial addition for anyone eating a plant-based diet.

A serving of 30g of walnuts has :

- ➤ 4.4g of protein

- ➤ 206 kcals (851 KJ)

- ➤ 20.6g of fat

- ➤ 2.2g of saturated fat

- ➤ 1.0g carbs

- ➤ 14.0g polyunsaturated fat

- ➤ 3.2g monounsaturated fat

- ➤ 1.4 g of fiber

- ➢ 135 mg of potassium

- ➢ 1.16 mg of vitamin E

- ➢ 1.4 g of fiber

- ➢ 135 mg of potassium

- ➢ 1.16 mg of vitamin E

Studies on animals indicate that walnuts are the richest nut in antioxidants, and may be helpful in the battle against cancer, particularly colon and breast cancer.

An eight-week study that followed 194 healthy adults who consumed 43 g of walnuts daily revealed that eating walnuts may benefit us and our gut microbes. The results showed an increase in beneficial gut bacteria, particularly those that produce butyrate. This short-chain fatty acid has anti-inflammatory and anti-cancer qualities, among other benefits.

2. Almonds:

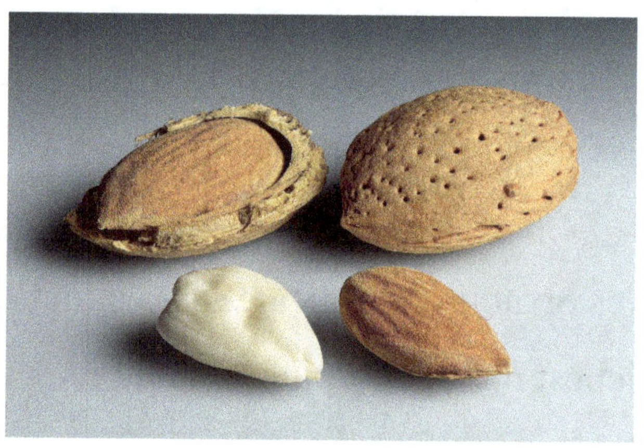

Might Aid in Weight Loss.

Although they are frequently referred to as nuts, almonds are the fruit of the almond tree and are teardrop-shaped edible seeds. You can purchase shelled or blanched, which treats shelled almonds with hot water to remove the outer brown coating and reveal the smooth, white interior.

Almonds have the highest calcium concentration of any nut; we need this mineral for strong bones and adequately operating our nerves and muscles. Almonds are also packed with heart-healthy monounsaturated fat, fiber, and vitamin E. Almonds' heart-healthy fat and high fiber content make it possible for them to lower cholesterol levels.

Eating almonds with the skin on may have even more advantages for gut health by encouraging the growth of Lactobacillus and Bifidobacteria, two good bacterial strains. Flavonoids, which are protective substances with antioxidant properties, are abundant in the skin. With about 4 g of fiber per 1-ounce serving, almonds rank among the nuts with the most amazing fiber content. The chance of developing diabetes, heart disease, and several types of cancer is also decreased by eating enough fiber. Moreover, fiber makes you feel full, which might aid in weight loss.

A 30g portion of almonds has :

- 184 calories and 760 kJ

- 6.3 g of protein

- 6.7 g of fat

- 1.3 g of fatty fat

- 11.5 g of monounsaturated fat

- 3.1 g of polyunsaturated fat

- 2.1 g of carbohydrates

- 2.2 g of fiber

- 72 mg of calcium

> 81 mg of magnesium

> Vitamin E: 7.19 mg

3. Cashews:

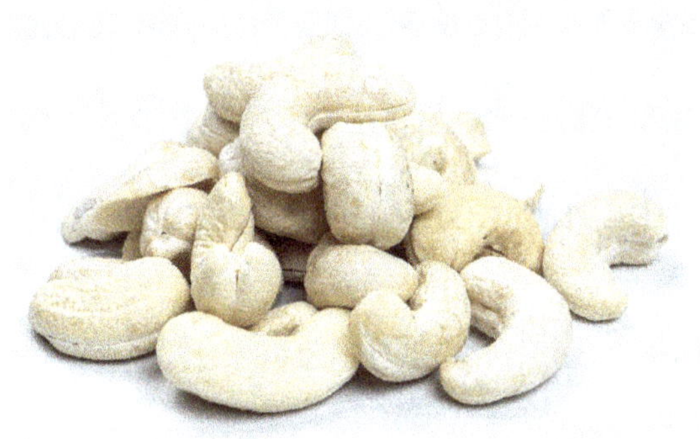

may aid in reducing "bad" cholesterol.

According to studies, consuming cashews may enhance blood lipid levels and lower blood pressure, which supports heart health.

Cashews are an excellent option for a vegetarian diet since they provide significant protein and are a valuable source of minerals like iron and zinc. Also, they contain a lot of magnesium, a mineral that may help with recollection and prevent age-related memory decline.

Cashews are a good source of plant sterols, which may help control cholesterol levels and heart-healthy monounsaturated fats.

30 grams of cashew nuts contain:

- 5.3 g of protein

- 14.5 g of fat

- 5.4g of carbohydrates

- 1.3g of fiber

- 2.9g of saturated fat

- 8.3g of monounsaturated fat

- 2.6g of polyunsaturated fat

- 81mg of magnesium

- 1.86mg of iron

- 1.77mg of zinc

- 172 kcal/712 KJ

4. Pecans:

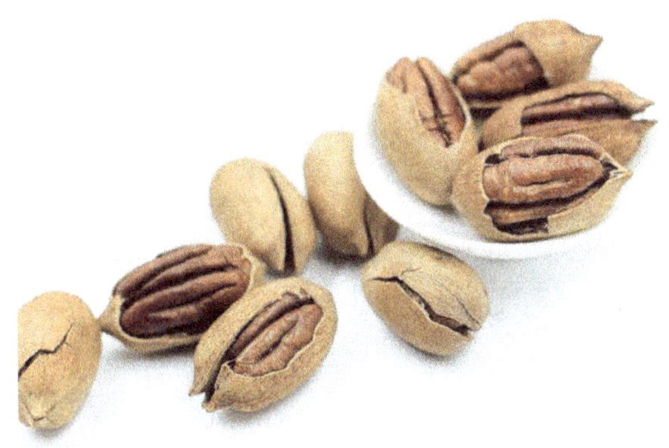

May Reduce Risk of Diabetes and Heart Disease.

Pecans can aid your heart health and be used to make delicious pies.

Plant sterols, powerful cholesterol-lowering agents, are abundant in heart-healthy pecans.

Pecans are also a good source of antioxidants, which aids in preventing plaque buildup that results in artery hardening. Moreover, they contain many oleic acids, a monounsaturated fat known for its heart-healthy properties in foods like avocados and olives.

A 30g serving of pecans provides:

- ➢ 207 kcals/853 KJ.

- ➢ 1.7g carbs

- ➢ 1.9g fiber

- ➢ 156 mg potassium

- ➢ 1.59mg zinc

- ➢ 2.8g protein

- ➢ 21.0g fat

- ➢ 1.7g saturated fat

- ➢ 12.8g monounsaturated fat

- ➢ 5.6g polyunsaturated fat

5. Brazil Nuts:

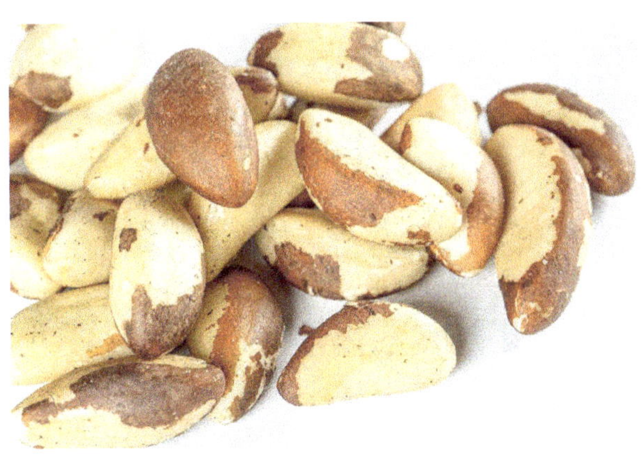

Protect Against Radicalization

Brazil nuts, which come from an Amazonian tree, are one of the highest food sources of the mineral selenium.

Selenium is a mineral that promotes immunity, works as a protective antioxidant, and speeds up the healing of wounds. We only need a minimal amount of Selenium.

Thus, you only need one to three Brazil nuts daily to meet your needs. Brazil nuts strengthen our defense mechanisms and assist in controlling blood cholesterol levels. They also contain vitamin E and the polyphenols gallic and ellagic acids.

30g of Brazil nuts contain the following nutrients:

- ➤ 205 calories/845 KJ

- ➤ 4.3 g of protein

- ➤ 20.5 g of fat

- ➤ 5.2 g of saturated fat

- ➤ 6.7 g of monounsaturated fat

- ➤ 7.6 g of polyunsaturated fat

- ➤ 0.9 g of carbs

- ➤ 51 mg of calcium;

- ➤ 123 mg of magnesium

- ➤ 1.7g of fiber

- ➤ Selenium, 76.2 mcg

6. Macadamia:

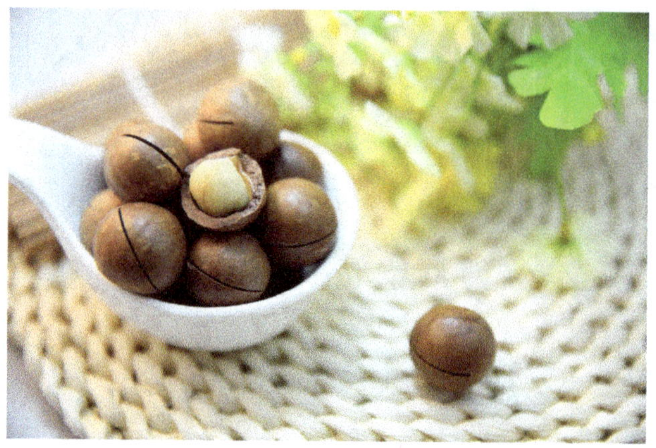

These nuts are loaded with good fats.

Macadamias have one of the highest fat contents and are frequently used in savory and sweet dishes to add flavor and texture.

Despite being notorious for having a lot of fat, macadamia nuts are not to be afraid of. These nuts contain the richest source of heart-healthy monounsaturated fats, and as a result, they aid in controlling cholesterol and heart disease risk factors.

They are a good source of fiber and contribute significantly to the intake of minerals, including magnesium, calcium, and potassium.

30 grams of macadamia nuts contain:

- ➢ 215 calories/901 KJ

- ➢ 2.4 grams of protein

- ➢ 22.7 grams of fat

- ➢ 17.7g monounsaturated fat

- ➢ 0.5g polyunsaturated fat

- ➢ 3.6g saturated fat

- ➢ 1.6g of carbohydrates

- ➢ 2.6g of fiber

- ➢ 110 mg of potassium

- ➤ 26 mg of calcium

- ➤ 39 mg of magnesium.

7. Pistachios:

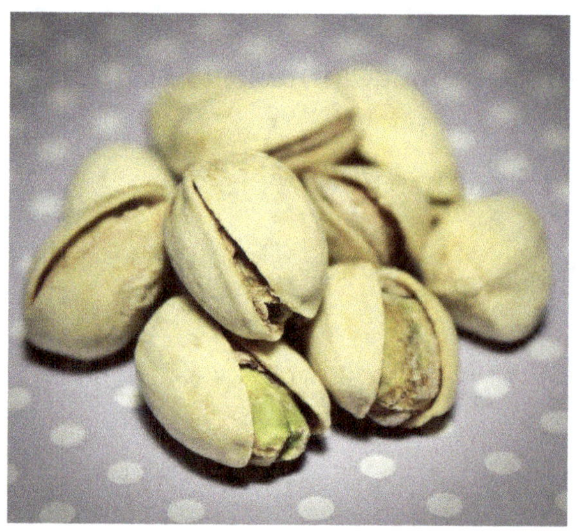

May Reduce Your Snacking.

Pistachios are a common element in puddings and sweets, and their fascinating color comes from pigments with antioxidant benefits.

Pistachios are the highest in potassium and have the lowest fat and calorie counts of most other nuts. They contain exceptionally high levels of phytosterols, which promote cardiovascular health.

Moreover, they are the only nut with adequate amounts of lutein and zeaxanthin, two antioxidants crucial for eye protection.

30g serving Pistachios contain:

> ➢ 6.1g of protein and

> ➢ 169 kcals/706 KJ

> ➢ 13.6 g of fat,

> ➢ 1.7 g of saturated fat

> ➢ 7.1 g of monounsaturated fat

> ➢ 4.1 g of polyunsaturated fat

- 5.4 g of carbs, 3.1 g of fiber

- 308 mg of potassium

- 1.18 mg of iron

- 1.37 mg of vitamin E

8. Hazelnuts:

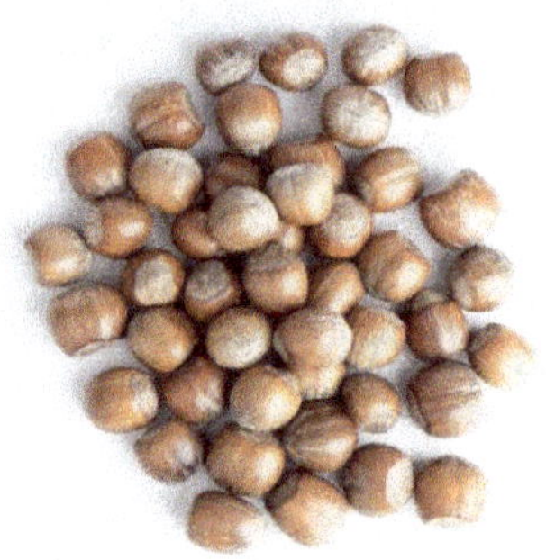

Aid in Chronic Disease Prevention.

Hazelnuts are the second-richest nut source of monounsaturated fat, which is good for the heart.

They are also anti-inflammatory and can aid with blood lipid management. They help boost vitamin E status because they are abundant in vitamins and minerals, especially in the elderly.

A nut that is generally healthful because of its high content of monounsaturated fats, which might enhance cardiovascular health and aid in the management of type 2 diabetes.

Also, they include several antioxidants that can help prevent chronic illnesses like cancer, heart disease, and inflammatory diseases.

The nutritional value of hazelnuts is as follows per 30g serving:

- ➤ 4.2g protein

- ➤ 19.1g fat

- ➤ 1.4g saturated fat

- ➤ 14.8g monounsaturated fat

- ➤ 2.0g polyunsaturated fat

- ➤ 1.8g carbs

- ➤ 2.1g fiber

- ➤ 219 mg potassium

- ➤ 22 mcg folate

9. Chestnuts

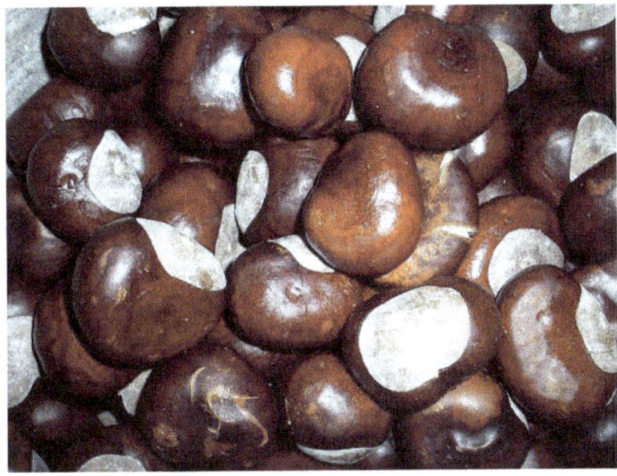

Chestnuts are a popular and adaptable ingredient low in fat and calories and a rich source of nourishing antioxidants.

Chestnuts are by far the lowest fat and calorie nut. They are also high in fiber and starchy carbohydrates, and when consumed raw, they are an excellent source of vitamin C.

Despite having less protein than other nuts, they can be ground to make gluten-free flour used in cakes and other baked goods.

30g of raw chestnuts supply the following nutrients:

- ➢ 59 kcal/246 KJ
- ➢ 0.5 g protein
- ➢ 3.1 g fat
- ➢ 0.1g saturated fat
- ➢ 0.1g monounsaturated fat
- ➢ 0.1g polyunsaturated fat
- ➢ 13.9 g carbs
- ➢ 1.5 g fiber
- ➢ 145 mg potassium

➢ 9 mg magnesium

➢ 17 mcg folate

➢ 12 mg vitamin C

10. Pine nuts:

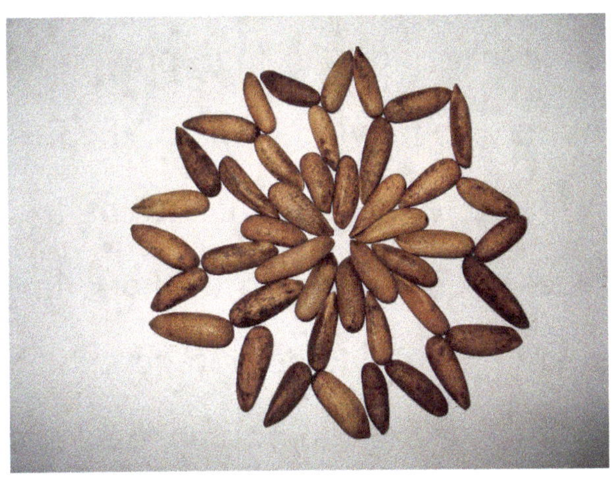

These tiny nuts give nutrition to salads, pasta, and dips and are a primary component of pesto. According to botany, pine nuts are seeds rather than nuts and come from many species of pine cones.

These nuts, exceptionally high in vitamin E, may maintain healthy skin and prevent aging by being included in the diet.

Pine nuts may help lower fasting blood glucose levels, and their high polyphenol content may help avoid some of the health issues related to diabetes, according to animal research. However, further clinical studies are required to comprehend the effects of foods high in polyphenols and how much should be consumed daily to attain these outcomes.

30g of pine nuts contain the following nutrients:

➤ 206 kcal/852 KJ

➤ 4.2 g of protein

➤ 20.6 g of fat

➤ 1.2 grams of carbs

➤ 0.8 grams of fiber

➤ 234 milligrams of potassium

➤ 81 milligrams of magnesium

➤ 4.16 milligrams of vitamin E

➤ 1.14 milligrams of vitamin B3

CHAPTER 4

CLASSIFICATION OF NUTS IN BASED ON PROTEIN CONTENT:

8 high-protein nuts you should eat

Recently, nuts have drawn much interest for their potential health advantages and capacity to prevent disease. As you browse the grocery store aisles, there are a variety of drinks, snacks, and spreads made with nuts and nut-based ingredients.

Nuts are typically a good source of heart-healthy lipids, vitamins, minerals, and antioxidants.

Yet, not all nuts have the same amount of nourishment. Some have a greater concentration of a specific nutrient than others.

The top eight nuts based on protein content are as follows:

1. Almond

With 1/4 cup (35 gram) serving of almonds, there are 7 grams of protein. In reality, almonds are seeds. Nonetheless, they are frequently grouped with nuts and considered high-protein food.

Almonds are rich in antioxidants in addition to being high in protein. These plant compounds shield the body against oxidative stress from free radicals, which can cause aging, heart disease, and cancer.

The most significant concentration of antioxidants is found in the brown skin layer surrounding almonds, so eating almonds with the skin is better for maximum health benefits.

Combine almonds with a piece of fruit to create a well-rounded snack.

2. walnut

There are 4.5 grams of protein in 1/4 cup (29 grams) of chopped walnuts.A fantastic method to increase your protein intake is by eating walnuts.

Moreover, walnuts contain heart-healthy lipids. Remarkably, they have more alpha-linolenic acid (ALA), an omega-3 fatty acid, than any other nut.

Some observational studies have associated decreased risk of heart disease with ALA intake.

Walnuts are a tasty addition to ground meats and can further boost the protein content of recipes using root because of their fatty texture and mouthfeel.

3. Pistachios

Have 6 grams of protein per 1/4 cup (30-gram) portion.

Pistachios have the same amount of protein as an egg in a serving. Compared to most other nuts, these nuts have a higher ratio of necessary amino acids to their protein composition.

Essential amino acids must be consumed in sufficient amounts through diet for the body to use them to create proteins necessary for vital processes.

Pistachios are enjoyed novelly by mixing them into nut butter and spreading it on toast, apples, or crackers.

4. Cashews

Each 1/4 cup (32 grams) of cashews has 5 grams of protein.

Technically, cashews are seeds. They have not only a lot of protein but also a lot of essential vitamins and minerals.

The Daily Value (DV) for copper is around 80% of a 1/4-cup (32-gram) serving. The mineral copper helps to make red blood cells and connective tissue and boosts immunity.

Studies have also linked low copper intake to an increased risk of osteoporosis, characterized by fragile bones.

5. Pine Nuts

For 1/4 cup (34 grams) of pine nuts, there are 4.5 grams of protein.

The seeds of some types of pine cones are known as pine nuts. Because of their high-fat content, they have a mild, sweet flavor and buttery texture that are highly regarded.

A 1/4-cup (34-gram) portion of pine nuts provides 23 grams of fat and 4 grams of protein.

Unsaturated fats comprise most of the fat in pine nuts, which may help lower heart disease risk factors. One of the pine nut's fatty acids may also have anti-inflammatory properties and help stop the spread of cancer.

Adding toasted pine nuts is a fantastic method to increase the protein content of salads, grain bowls, or vegetables. Cook pine nuts in a skillet over medium heat until aromatic, about a few minutes.

6. Brazil nuts

Protein: 4.75 grams per serving of 1/4 cup (33 grams). Brazil nuts are the largest in a bag of mixed nuts and are made from the seeds of a rainforest tree, and are simple to identify.

They offer protein, good fats, fiber, and various vitamins. Moreover, one of the best nutritional sources of Selenium, a crucial element that supports thyroid function and shields the body from infection, is found in Brazil nuts.

Selenium is only one Brazil nut (5 grams) and is over 175% of the DV.

For a protein-rich trail mix, try combining Brazil nuts with other nuts and seeds, dried mango, and bits of dark chocolate.

7. peanut

A serving of 1/4 cup (37 grams) of peanuts has 9.5 grams of protein.

Despite being a legume, peanuts are considered nuts from a dietary and culinary perspective.

They offer a significant amount of plant-based protein like other legumes do. Peanuts contain the most protein of any regularly eaten nut.

Moreover, peanuts are among the best food sources of biotin, a vitamin that aids in the body's ability to turn food into valuable energy. Combine peanut butter and bananas or layer them on toast for a well-rounded snack with protein, lipids, and carbohydrates.

8. Hazelnuts

For 1/4 cup (34 grams) serving, there are 5 grams of protein. Hazelnuts are a delicious source of protein because of their somewhat sweet, buttery, and toasted flavor.

According to studies, including hazelnuts in your diet may help lower LDL (bad) cholesterol and raise HDL (good) cholesterol, reducing your chance of developing heart disease.

Make your own "Nutella" spread for a high-protein snack. 2 scoops (60 grams) of chocolate protein powder, 1 tablespoon (6 grams) of cocoa powder, and 2 tablespoons (30 mL) of maple syrup are blended with 1 cup (135 grams) of hazelnuts.

The healthiest and worst types of nut to consume:

Nuts to avoid for your diet:

Macadamia and pecan nuts

Macadamia nuts (10–12 nuts; 2–21 grams of fat; 3–20 grams of protein) and pecans (18–20 halves; 3–20 grams of fat) have the most calories per ounce (200 each), the least amount of protein, and the fattest.

They're still good nuts, though: Only 40 calories per ounce separate these nuts from the lowest-calorie nuts.

Any form of raw, plain nut will provide you with an appropriate dosage of healthful fats and nutrients, as long as you're practicing sensible portion control and refraining from eating handfuls at a time.

Heart-healthiest nuts

Walnuts

All nuts, including walnuts, have heart-healthy omega-3 fats, but walnuts have a lot of ALA (ALA). A 2006 Spanish study found that walnuts were as effective as olive oil at reducing inflammation and oxidation in the arteries after consuming a fatty meal. Research has revealed that ALA may assist heart arrhythmias.

The brain's healthiest nuts

Peanuts

Peanuts, technically are legumes but more commonly referred to as nuts, are rich in folate, a vitamin crucial for brain growth that may guard against cognitive decline.

This makes peanuts a fantastic choice for vegetarians, who may be deficient in folate, and expectant mothers who require folate to prevent their unborn children from birth abnormalities.

Peanuts, like the majority of other nuts, are rich in vitamin E and good fats that support the brain. Peanuts provide 28 unshelled nuts per ounce, which amounts to 170 calories, 7 grams of protein, and 14 grams of fat.

Men's best nuts

Brazil and pecan nuts

Creamy Selenium, a mineral that may guard against diseases like prostate cancer, is abundant in Brazil nuts. Eat these foods cautiously because one nut carries more than a day's worth of calories.

The risk of type 2 diabetes may be increased, according to recent studies. Brazil nuts have 6 per ounce and provide 190 calories, 19 grams of fat, and 4 grams of protein.

Pecans also benefit men's health. They contain high amounts of beta-sitosterol, a plant steroid that may aid with benign prostatic hyperplasia (BPH) or symptoms of an enlarged prostate. 18 to 20 halves of pecans make up one ounce, which has roughly 200 calories, 21 grams of fat, and 3 grams of protein.

The best nuts for preventing disease

Almonds

Almonds are a fantastic food for overall health since they have more calcium than any other nut and are relatively low in calories.

Moreover, they are high in fiber and vitamin E, an antioxidant that protects against harmful inflammation and may help prevent diseases like lung cancer and age-related cognitive decline. Since they can be eaten raw, toasted, slivered, or coated with various tasty flavors, such as Wasabi & Soy Sauce or Lime 'n Chili, almonds are frequently a favorite among nut lovers.

Nuts that are ideal for chocolate lovers

Choose almonds that have been sprinkled with cocoa:

Keep it simple with Emeralds Cocoa Roast Almonds rather than burying your nuts beneath a thick layer of sugary chocolate candy, like Jordan almonds or peanut M&Ms.

These nuts include 150 calories, 13 grams of fat, and 1 gram of sugar per ounce and are delicately powdered with cocoa powder and sweetened with sucralose.

But, anything more chocolate than nut should be considered confectionery rather than a way to meet your recommended daily intake of good fats.

The ideal nuts for a sweet tooth

Give natural glazed nuts a try.

Do you want something sweet and satiating without the added calories and high-fructose corn syrup?

Go no further than Sahale Snacks' glazed nuts, available in flavors including Cashews with Pomegranate and Vanilla (160 calories, 11 grams of fat, and 5 grams of protein per ounce) and Almonds with Cranberries, Honey, and Sea Salt (150 calories, 10 grams fat, 4 grams protein per ounce).

They include only 6 grams of sugar per ounce and are sweetened with organic cane juice and tapioca syrup. But watch out not to consume the entire bag!

Suitable nuts for salt cravings

Try to find "lightly salted" peanuts.

A handful or two of salted nuts daily will only harm you if you have high blood pressure or your doctor has advised you to avoid salt for other reasons. Of course, unsalted nuts are also an option. But to fulfill a salty appetite without going overboard, search for intermediate varieties like Fantastic Pistachios Lightly Salted or Planters Lightly Salted Peanuts, Almonds, and Cashews (45-55 mg sodium) (80 mg). Also, look at the ingredient labels: Some brands have less salt than others, such as Back to Nature Salted Almonds (75 mg sodium).

To sum up:

A good source of plant-based protein is nuts. In addition to adding them to numerous foods to increase their protein value, they make an easy snack.

Most of the protein per serving is found in peanuts, although all the nuts on this list are good protein providers.

Cashews, hazelnuts, and Brazil nuts are intriguing alternatives if you cannot consume peanuts or want to try other protein-rich nuts.

CHAPTER 5

HOW TO INCORPORATE NUTS AND SEED PRODUCTS INTO YOUR DIET

Now that you know the various nuts' health benefits, paying attention to how you consume them is critical to reaping the most significant health rewards.

Due to their ability to slow down digestion and the breakdown of sugar, nuts are a fantastic food to eat after consuming a carbohydrate such as fruit or juice.

There are numerous strategies to increase the number of nuts in your diet, including:

> - A yogurt parfait is a great place to add chopped walnuts.

- Make your almond butter, a popular substitute for peanut butter, by grinding your almonds.

- Prepare banana nut bread from scratch.

- Pecans can be added to a salad.

- When preparing vegetable stir-fries, use cashew nuts.

- Use almonds in a protein shake containing a banana and milk.

- To make a Mediterranean-style salad, combine with feta cheese, olives, and chopped almonds.

- Make a paste of herbs and walnuts for a grilled chicken to use as a garnish.

➤ Have a handful of raw or dry-roasted nuts as a snack instead of a biscuit or cake.

➤ Mix nuts and seeds with dishes that are low in calories (such as vegetables). It is a tasty method to improve vegetable-based foods, such as Asian-style dishes or salads.

➤ Nuts and seeds are a fantastic protein substitute for meats, fish, and eggs if you're vegan or vegetarian. They also have niacin, iron, zinc, and fat. You might require more than 30 grams of nuts and seeds daily to get enough protein.

➤ Consume them alongside foods high in vitamin C and mix them into juices like tomato, capsicum, orange, and citrus to increase your body's ability to absorb iron.

➤ Unless you favor the flavor and texture of soaked nuts, there is no need to wash or remove the skin from nuts (or "activate" them). In actuality, nuts' skin contains a lot of phytochemicals with anti-inflammatory and antioxidant capabilities.

➤ Roasting nuts (dry or in oil) improves their flavor but doesn't significantly change how much fat they contain. Due to their physical density, nuts cannot absorb much oil, even when submerged. Nuts typically absorb just 2% of additional fat

➢ Due to their higher sodium level, salted nuts should be avoided, especially if you have high blood pressure. Make raw and unsalted roasted nuts your go-to daily, and save salted nuts for special occasions.

optimum trail mix

Dried fruit, seeds, and raw nuts:

There are various brands and variations of trail mix to choose from. If the nuts are roasted, search for "dry roasted" rather than "oil roasted" or for a trail mix containing raw nuts. Nuts go well with fruit, seeds, and possibly even a little dark chocolate;

nevertheless, it's essential to consider the calories and to serve size.

CHAPTER 6

WHAT HAPPENS TO YOUR BODY IF YOU EAT NUTS DAILY:

You might be curious about what happens to your body when you consume nuts regularly, even if specific varieties have more nutrients than others. And should you consume specific nuts more or less frequently than others?

1. Almonds, peanuts, pecans, and walnuts:

Eating each five times a week dramatically lowered their LDL ("bad") cholesterol levels.

2. You might enhance your LDL, HDL, and total cholesterol levels:

Also, consuming walnuts, pistachios, and hazelnuts may help increase "good" HDL cholesterol levels. According to research, nuts' phytosterols, a class of lipids, may be to blame for lowering LDL levels. The same analysis noted that the highest phytosterols could be found in pistachios, pine nuts, and almonds.

Also, it was shown that eating almonds, walnuts, pecans, and peanuts lower overall cholesterol levels.

3. Increase your antioxidant intake:

Flavonoids are chemicals naturally present in plant-based diets and are known to be present in nuts, including almonds. They are not only abundant in antioxidants, but they may also be able to shield you from free radicals that could cause atherosclerosis, a hardening of the blood arteries, and a rise in your risk of heart disease.

4.You may consume more antioxidants while eating certain types of nuts.

The highest concentrations of tocopherol, a vitamin E form that is also an antioxidant linked to a lowered risk of cancer and inflammation, are found in cashews and almonds.

5. You might shed some pounds:

According to research, nuts like tree nuts and peanuts do not increase your risk of becoming obese. According to a 2019 study from Nutrition Research, eating more than one to two servings of nuts per week may be associated with a lower risk of weight gain, overweight, and obesity. Protein and fiber, which boost feelings of fullness and decrease appetite, may cause this phenomenon.

Due to changed hunger sensitivity and management, other research also found that consuming nuts could not always result in weight loss, particularly for people who are overweight or obese.

6. You could lower your risk of developing colon cancer:

Nuts have anti-inflammatory and antioxidant qualities that may lessen the risk of tumor development. However, including nuts in a balanced diet is only sometimes harmful to other potential health advantages (as long as you are not allergic).

7. You could consume more sodium:

Although nuts are healthy, how they are prepared certainly counts. The salt content in roasted salted or flavoring nuts can be significant. Too much sodium can increase blood pressure and your risk of heart attack, stroke, and other cardiovascular diseases.

However, it may not be a good idea to rely solely on nuts to control your weight as there are many other aspects to consider, including the kinds and portions of food you eat, your genetics, how active you are, and more. Failure, If you are watching your sodium intake, have high blood pressure or have diabetes, try to choose unsalted nuts.

8. Certain micronutrients may be consumed in excess:

Excessive consumption of some nuts, particularly Brazil nuts, can eventually cause selenosis, sometimes called selenium intoxication. Of all nut varieties, Brazil nuts have the highest concentration of Selenium, with each gram providing 35 micrograms, or roughly two-thirds, of the recommended daily intake. So, just one to two nuts per day already satisfy the RDA, while a 1-ounce dose of nuts has 544 micrograms of Selenium or almost 989% of the RDA.

 The recommended daily intake for Selenium is 400 micrograms as a point of reference. Consuming more may lead to risks of developing selenium intoxication symptoms like weakness, exhaustion, and burning or prickling sensations

CHAPTER 7:

TIPS FOR STORING NUTS

Are Nuts Perishable?

Indeed, nuts of all varieties can become deficient. The nuts' lipids and nutrients will deteriorate when exposed to air, hot temperatures, and light. Moisture will hasten disintegration and promote the development of germs and mold.

The leading causes of poor nuts are:

• **Rancidity:** When nuts' fats degrade, they turn rancid. Nuts quickly turn rotten when exposed to heat and air.

• **Pests:** Nuts are a favorite food of pantry moths. Rodents getting into people's nut storage is a concern for some individuals.

Learn how to mouse-proof your food storage and prevent and get rid of pantry pests.

• **Mold:** Nuts are susceptible to the growth of molds, which create aflatoxins as byproducts. These substances can harm the liver and are cancer-causing. Lung irritation from inhaling aflatoxins is another possibility. High moisture levels mainly cause mold growth in nuts.

• **Bacteria:** Besides mold, harmful bacteria can occasionally grow on nuts. Nuts have been connected to outbreaks of listeria and salmonella.

• **Taking in fragrances:** Nuts occasionally take in the smells of meals that are stored nearby. Although they are still safe to consume, because of this, the taste is affected. Never keep nuts next to cleaning supplies or chemicals.

How to Store Nuts Properly

You can store nuts with or without their shells. They will survive longer if you keep them in the cover, but shelling them beforehand will make them simpler to grip and utilize.

Thus, it's a matter of taste. In either case, keeping your nuts hydrated is crucial by storing them in an airtight container. Even a freezer bag made of plastic will work.

Unlike shelled nuts, nuts in their shell generally survive 20–50% longer.

Keep your nuts away from foods with intense flavors like onions to retain their quality. They have the propensity to absorb smells from their surroundings. Shelled nuts can be kept for three months at room temperature.

Nuts can be held in the freezer for a year or more or in the refrigerator for up to six months. So that you know which nuts to use first, mark the packages of your nuts with the date they were placed in storage.

If they taste stale, roast your nuts for 10 minutes at 350 degrees. These will restore their flavor. Nut oils cannot be salvaged once they have deteriorated. But as long as you adhere to these storage recommendations, you should never experience that issue.

How to Preserve Nuts for a Long Time

In general, nuts are only an excellent food to store for a short time. They will still get rotten even under perfect storage conditions.

Nuts should be stored for up to two years, only gather as many supplies as you can rotate through this time.

If you wish to keep nuts for at least two years, you must employ one of these techniques.

Freezer:

The simplest way to keep nuts for a long time is like this. The low temperature inhibits the formation of mold and oxidation. The nuts should still be placed in an airtight bag or vacuum-sealed container before guarding against oxygen and moisture.

Root Cellar:

Unshelled nuts can be kept in root cellars for up to a year. The root cellar's low temperature preserves the nuts.

Humidity is one issue with storing nuts in a root cellar, though. Most root cellars need a humidity level of roughly 80% to keep fruits fresh. Contrarily, nuts require a humidity of

57% to 70%. This room humidity will maintain the nutmeat's optimal humidity level of 4-8% (hazelnuts and macadamia nuts need higher humidity).

Consider designing a separate space with humidity controls if you intend to store a lot of nuts in your root cellar. Store the nuts in bins that are rodent-proof and well-ventilated.

Airtight Containers with Oxygen Absorbers:

Iron packets called oxygen absorbers take oxygen out of the air. An oxygen-free storage environment is produced when the nuts are placed in an airtight, tightly closed container, like a Mylar bag.

The nuts will live much longer than if stored without oxygen absorbers, but they will eventually go wrong, especially if stored at high temperatures. Although it varies, most nuts, when kept in this manner at room temperature, should keep for around two years.

Keep in Honey

You can put a few nuts in honey jars if you need to store a few nuts. Nuts can be stored in honey for over two years without going bad since honey is a natural preservative that never goes bad, even at room temperature.

preserving in syrup

Nuts can also be preserved for a long time by being canned in sugar syrup. A natural preservative is sugar. Furthermore, canning helps remove oxygen and makes the jar's lid airtight.

Conclusion

Eating a range of nuts is generally advised because each nut type provides a specific number and type of nutrients. But, as mentioned above, consuming Brazil nuts is moderate, and less frequently is recommended to prevent selenium intoxication.

Furthermore, the quantity of nuts you consume affects you. Although nuts contain heart-healthy lipids, they are also high in calories. The protein you need may vary depending on your age and calorie requirements.

One tablespoon of nut butter, 12 almonds, 24 pistachios, 7 walnut halves, or 1 serving of protein is all acceptable substitutes.

Compared to those who consume just one serving per week, which decreases the risk by 4%, consuming one serving of nuts per day may reduce the risk of heart disease by 27%.

Eating a range of nuts and seeds can offer several health advantages. But remember to incorporate them into your diet in moderation as part of a balanced one.

Nutritional value: Nuts and seeds are a good source of several nutrients, including fiber, vitamins, minerals, healthy fats, and protein.

One ounce of almonds, for instance, has 6 grams of protein, 14 grams of beneficial fats, and 3.5 grams of fiber and is a vital source of magnesium and vitamin E.

They have several health advantages that have been linked to their consumption. For instance, studies indicate that including nuts and seeds in a balanced diet may lower the chance of developing heart disease, diabetes, and particular types of cancer. Moreover, nuts and seeds may enhance cognitive performance and reduce the risk of cognitive decline brought on by aging.

Weight loss: Contrary to what many think, nuts and seeds may help with weight management. According to research, nuts, and seeds can help you manage your appetite, consume fewer calories, and lose weight more effectively.

Allergies: Although nuts and seeds provide many health advantages, some people may experience life-threatening allergic responses. One of the most prevalent and potentially fatal food allergies is an allergy to nuts. If you have a nut allergy, avoiding all nuts is crucial, and ask a healthcare provider for suggestions on safe substitutes.

Preparation: Nuts and seeds can be prepared and eaten raw, roasted, or as nut butter. To avoid unnecessary salt and additional oils, search for unsalted and unroasted versions of nuts and seeds while shopping. Nut butter shouldn't contain any other sugars or fats. Nuts and seeds should be stored correctly to avoid rotting in a cold, dry environment.

Nuts are a highly flexible snack with fantastic protein, healthy fats, and vital fiber sources. Whatever your taste, there is a

delicious nut out there for you!

www.ingramcontent.com/pod-product-compliance
Lightning Source LLC
Chambersburg PA
CBHW061555250726
48657CB00021B/1745